M000029019

MARY JANE'S PASSPORT

By: David Taborga

ISBN: 978-0-578-50040-9 (Paperback)

Any reference to historical events, real people, or real places are used fictitiously. Names, characters, and places are products of the authors imagination.

Written and illustrated by David Taborga

Cochino, Inc, in the United States of America

First Printed Edition 2019.
www.TheCochino.com

Acknowledgments

I first want to acknowledge and thank my incredibly strong and beautiful wife, Lynn, for putting up with all the craziness and helping me overcome the hurdles that came along with this project. My family and friends have given me nothing but encouragement from the very beginning - thank you, and I love you. Also, I want to give a big thank you to my colleagues in the Maryland medical cannabis industry, who have demonstrated a passion for cannabis that is unrivaled. I couldn't have completed this book without you all. Thank you.

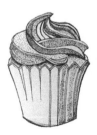

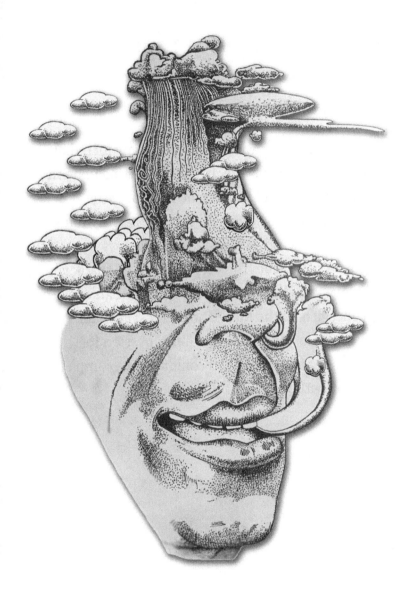

"Mendo Breath" Detail

Contents

Introduction 9

Types of Cannabis.. 10

Cannabinoids 11

Power of Edibles.. 17

Terpenes and the Entourage Effect 21

Sativa Notes... 25

Indica Notes 41

Hybrid Notes.. 57

About the Author... 72

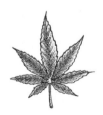

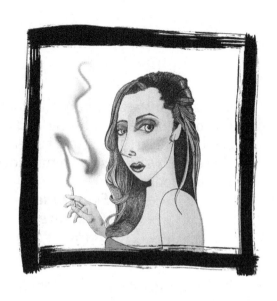

I am bold, confident, resilient, unapologetic and
most important of all, I am all-natural. I
help soothe the soul and alleviate the pain.
I'm always there when you need me.
I am Mary Jane.

#endthestigma

Types of Cannabis

Sativa
DAYTIME:
MIND / HIGH

Sativa strains are traditionally known for their energetic, uplifting, and great cerebral effects. This strain is great for those that want to stay on the move and be productive.

-Sour Diesel
-Jack Herer
-Durban Poison

Indica
NIGHTIME:
BODY / STONED

Indica strains are usually more sedating with full-body effects. Those who seek a relaxing nightcap tend to use this strain later in the evening.

-Northern Lights
-Blue Cheese
-Hindu Kush

Hybrid

Hybrid strains offer the best of both worlds with a combination effect from both Sativa and Indica. Many hybrid strains will be well balanced, or either Indica or Sativa dominate.

-White Widow
-Pineapple Express
-Chemdawg

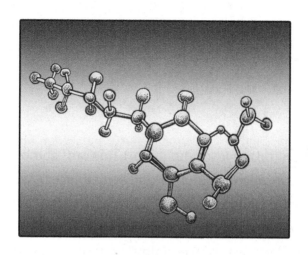

Cannabinoids

The cannabis plant naturally produces a particular class of chemical compounds. Cannabinoids can interact with receptors in our cells, altering the release of chemicals in the brain. These unique compounds can produce a wide array of effects throughout the body.

Disclaimer! The information given throughout this book about cannabinoids and terpenes is strictly about the chemical compounds naturally produced by the cannabis plant and not produced synthetically.

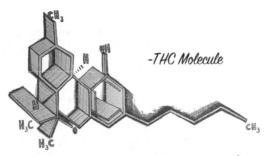

-THC Molecule

THC- (tetrahydrocannabinol) This cannabinoid is one of the most popular and sought after chemical compounds in cannabis. THC delivers very heavy psychoactive effects usually resulting in euphoric highs. Contingent on certain strains and varying concentrations of THC, this cannabinoid can bring forth feelings of peace and tranquility while others may experience an increase in anxiety levels.

Medical Benefits
* Pain reliever   * Anti-inflammatory
* Anti-oxidant * Eliminates nausea
* Treats mental health conditions
* Improves creativity   * Appetite stimulant
* Euphoric effects   * Treats digestive health issues

Potential Side Effects
* Dry mouth   * Dizziness   * Increased appetite
* Memory impairment   * Paranoia/Anxiety

THCA- (tetrahydrocannabinolic acid) This cannabinoid is found in abundance in raw and live cannabis. Heat can quickly convert THCA into the psychoactive cannabinoid THC by a process known as decarboxylation. Decarboxylation is the term that describes what occurs when you smoke, vaporize or cook cannabis flower.

THCA > > THC

Research efforts are ongoing with THCA and many other cannabinoids, but right now evidence suggests that THCA can offer many medical benefits without the psychoactive effects of its more popular counterpart THC.

Medical Benefits
* Anti-inflammatory properties
* Neuroprotective properties help with neurodegenerative diseases.
* Anti-nausea
* Appetite stimulant
* Insomnia

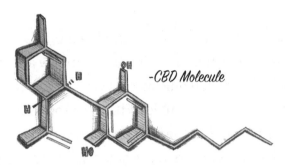
-CBD Molecule

CBD- (cannabidiol) This cannabinoid is a popular one for those who do not seek the intoxicating effects of THC but instead still seek the benefits from its medical applications. While clinical trials are still ongoing with CBD, evidence has shown relief in dealing with depression, body pain, epilepsy, and insomnia. CBD can influence a wide range of receptors in the body and the brain. CBD influences the way THC interacts with CB1 receptors in your endocannabinoid system. CBD will affect how high THC will make you feel.

Medical Benifets
* Anti-tumor   * Neuroprotective properties
* Epilepsy   * Depression/Anxiety
* Anti-Inflammatory   * Pain reliever
* Mental Disorders/Schizophrenic

CBN- (Cannabinol) This cannabinoid can be found in abundance in older flower. Time and bad storage practices can speed up the gradual breakdown of **THCA** into **CBN**. This cannabinoid is very soothing and sedative when combined with THC. Be wary of any old cannabis flower found; you could be in for a harsh smoke and early nap.

CBG- (Cannabigerol) is the lesser-known cannabinoid in cannabis. This cannabinoid is non-psychoactive but still carries many medicinal benefits. Believe it or not, both THC and CBD come from CBG in the early stages of the cannabis plant. Although this cannabinoid is not present in large quantities in most strains, it is still out there. Breeders are currently experimenting with cross breeding and the manipulation of genetics to help give this cannabinoid greater dominance.

Medical Benefits
* Anti-bacterial   * Anti-depressant
* Neuroprotective effects   * Powerful vasodilator

CBC- (Cannabichromene) Similar to CBG, this cannabinoid gets very little praise or attention, yet has many medical benefits. CBC is found in higher concentrations in younger plants. CBC has the same ancestry as both THC and CBD in that they are all rooted from cannabigerolic acid (CBGA). It is non-psychoactive yet carries a wide range of benefits. Finding products with an abundance of CBC can be challenging. With more research and more exposure in the cannabis market, this cannabinoid could be very impactful in modem medicine.

Medical Benifets
* Anti-Microbial   * Anti-Inflammatory
* Analgesic   * Anti-Depressant   * Migraines
* Anti-tumor   * Sedative effects

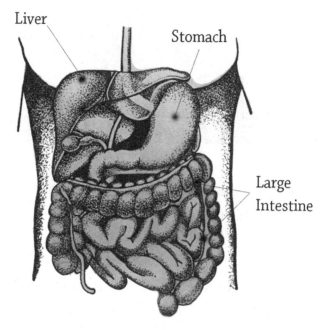

Liver

Stomach

Large
Intestine

Power of Edibles

Edibles introduce cannabinoids through the
digestive system. Eating edibles allows THC to be
absorbed through the intestinal tracts slowly. The
next process involves the liver, which breaks down
THC and converts it into a more potent chemical
called 11-hydroxy-THC (11-OH-THC). Once this
new chemical compound is made, it is released into
the bloodstream. This results in very intense
psychoactive effects that last much longer.

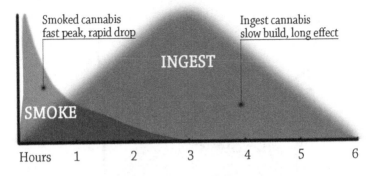

Smoked cannabis
fast peak, rapid drop

Ingest cannabis
slow build, long effect

INGEST

SMOKE

Hours   1   2   3   4   5   6

-Smoking cannabis gives instant effects but tends to last in the 2-3 hour range.

-Edibles bind to fats in the body, allowing the effects to last much longer than other methods. The effects usually last 4-6 hours but can fluctuate depending on the dosage.

-Body chemistry, metabolism, body weight, and dosage amounts all factor into your experience with edibles.

-Always start low at the beginning then adjust dosages accordingly the next day.

-Remember! Edibles can sneak up on you. Set time- 40 min to 1 hour and a half.

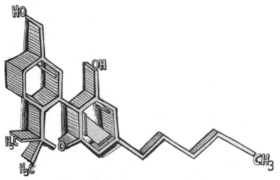

11-Hydroxy-THC

11-Hydroxy-THC is believed to be four to five times more psychoactive than THC, so consume with caution. Remember! Start with a low amount and adjust accordingly.

5mg	Micro dosage: mild effects and relief from pain, stress, and anxiety.
10-15mg	Good starting point: brings euphoria and muscle relaxation.
15-30mg	Moderate-high tolerance: a medical patient with developed tolerances.
30-60mg	For experienced users only: may impair coordination and alter perception.
60-90+mg	Very high tolerance: patients with cancer and other ailments that require higher dosages.

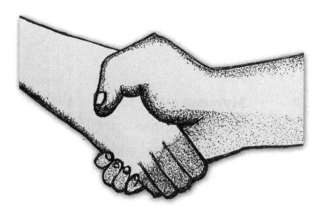

Terpenes
and the Entourage Effect

The essential oils of plants are what gives it's distinctive aroma and taste profiles to all organic matter. Throughout history, humans have used essential oils in a wide variety of products - from soaps to pharmaceuticals. Terpenes from cannabis offer many medical benefits when it joins forces with cannabinoids THC/CBD, and this is what many refer to as " The Entourage Effect." The relationship between the two provides a vast spectrum of therapeutic effects. When shopping for strains, patients should always take into account which terpene profile is present to better achieve the desired results.

Terpene List

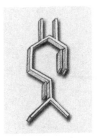

Myrcene can be found in abundance in mangos and also hops. This terpene is a great sleep aid and muscle relaxant. Aromas: Pungent, flowers, and earthy.

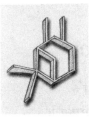

Pinene can be found in pine needles. Gives a sense of alertness. Anti-inflammatory and anti-bacterial properties. Aromas: Earthy, pine.

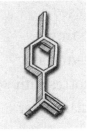

Limonene can be found in citrus fruits. Gives a happy euphoric high. Anti-anxiety, anti-deppression. Aromas: Citrus, fresh spice.

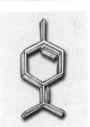

Terpinolene, found in coriander. Anti-oxidant, anti-bacterial. A very sedative terpene. Aromas: Pine, herbal, lime.

Terpene List

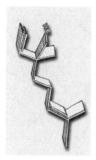 **Linalool** commonly found in lavender and coriander. Helps to reduce stress. Anti-anxiety, analgesic, relaxant, sedative, and anti-depressant. Aroma: Lavender, flowers, fresh spice.

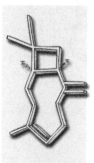 **Caryophyllene** is known to be a spicy, peppery terpene. Found in black pepper, cloves, and cinnamon. Has anti-inflammatory, and anti-anxiety properties. Aroma: Spice, citrus.

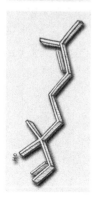 **Humulene** can be found in hops, basil, and cloves. This terpene carries an earthy aroma. Known to suppress the appetite. Anti-bacterial, anti-inflammatory. Aroma: Floral, hops.

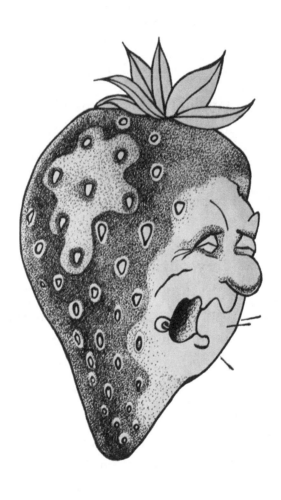

"Strawberry Cough" Detail

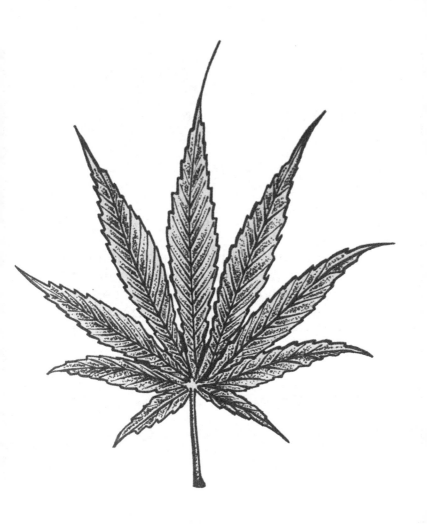

Sativa
Energy, Uplifting,
Cerebral, Creativity, Focus, Head High

Sour Diesel

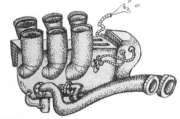

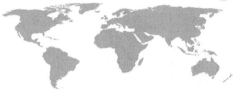

This very stimulating Sativa strain named for its super pungent, fuel-like aroma offers an uplifting cerebral high. It is great at combating depression, anxiety, and pain, and is also very energizing.

Cultivator... _____

Method... 🌸 Flower ⭕   💧 Concentrate ⭕

THC% _____   🧁 Edible ⭕

CBD% _____

Top 3 Terpenes... _____
_____
_____

Notes: _____
_____
_____

Strain

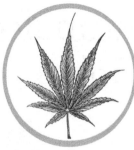

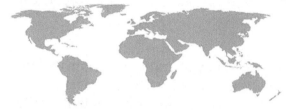

Cultivator... _____

Method... Flower ◯   Concentrate ◯

THC% ____   Edible ◯

CBD% ____

Top 3 Terpenes... _____
_____
_____

Notes: _____
_____
_____

Acapulco Gold

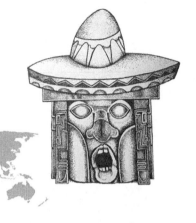

This is a very well-known strain that originated in the Acapulco areas of Mexico. Its orange hairs resemble a golden nugget. An aroma of burnt toffee lingers when the bud is broken up.

Cultivator... _____

Method... Flower O   Concentrate O

THC% ____   Edible O

CBD% ____

Top 3 Terpenes... _____
_____
_____

Notes: _____
_____
_____

_____

Strain

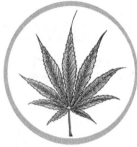

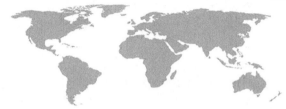

Cultivator... _____

Method... ![flower] Flower ⭕   ![drop] Concentrate ⭕

THC% ____   ![cupcake] Edible ⭕

CBD% ____

Top 3 Terpenes... _____
_____
_____

Notes: _____
_____
_____

Strawberry Cough

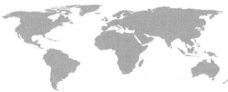
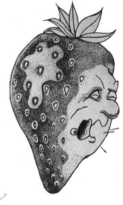

This strain may help manage social anxieties and stress. It has a sweet smell of fresh strawberries and offers uplifting and euphoric effects.

Cultivator...

Method...   Flower O   Concentrate O

THC% _____   Edible O

CBD% _____

Top 3 Terpenes...

Notes:

_____

Strain

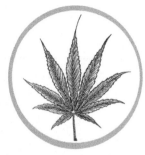

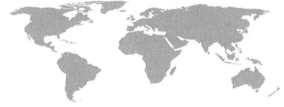

_____

Cultivator... _____

Method... 🌸 Flower ⭘   💧 Concentrate ⭘

THC% ____   🧁 Edible ⭘

CBD% ____

Top 3 Terpenes... _____
_____
_____

Notes: _____
_____
_____

_____

Strain

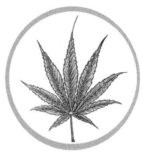

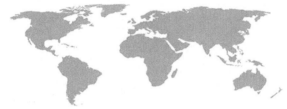

_____

Cultivator... _____

Method... Flower O   Concentrate O

THC% ____   Edible O

CBD% ____

Top 3 Terpenes... _____
_____
_____

Notes: _____
_____
_____

_____

Strain

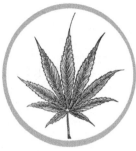

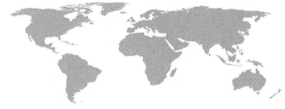

Cultivator... _____

Method... Flower ⭕ Concentrate ⭕

THC% ____ Edible ⭕

CBD% ____

Top 3 Terpenes... _____
_____
_____

Notes: _____
_____
_____

_____

Strain

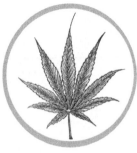

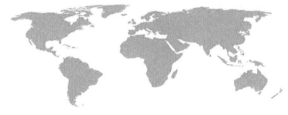

_____

Cultivator... _____

Method... Flower **O**   Concentrate **O**

THC% ____   Edible **O**

CBD% ____

Top 3 Terpenes... _____
_____
_____

Notes: _____
_____
_____

_____

Strain

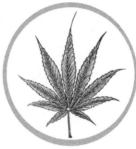

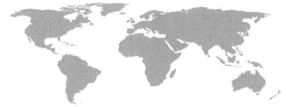

Cultivator... _____

Method... 🌸 Flower ⭕   💧 Concentrate ⭕

THC% ____   🧁 Edible ⭕

CBD% ____

Top 3 Terpenes... _____
_____
_____

Notes: _____
_____
_____

_____

Strain

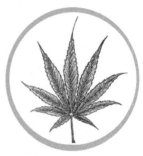

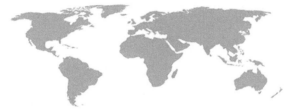

_____

Cultivator... _____

Method... 🌸 Flower ⭕ 💧 Concentrate ⭕

THC% ____ 🧁 Edible ⭕

CBD% ____

Top 3 Terpenes... _____
_____
_____

Notes: _____
_____
_____

Strain

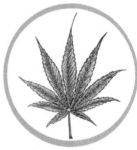

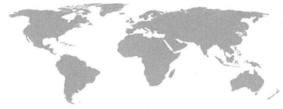

Cultivator... _____

Method... Flower ⭕   Concentrate ⭕

THC% ____   Edible ⭕

CBD% ____

Top 3 Terpenes... _____
_____
_____

Notes: _____
_____
_____

_____

Strain

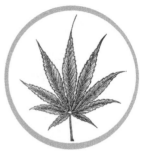

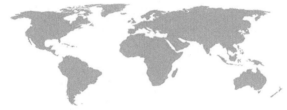

_____

Cultivator... _____

Method... 🌸 Flower ⭕   💧 Concentrate ⭕

THC% _____   🧁 Edible ⭕

CBD% _____

Top 3 Terpenes... _____
_____
_____

Notes: _____
_____
_____

Strain

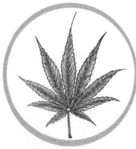

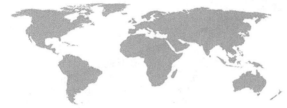

Cultivator... _____

Method... Flower **O**   Concentrate **O**

THC% ____   Edible **O**

CBD% ____

Top 3 Terpenes...
_____
_____
_____

Notes:
_____
_____
_____

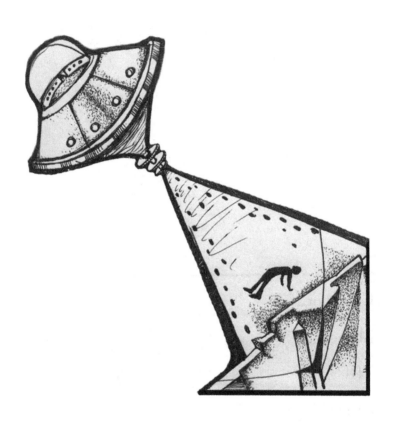

"Northern Lights" Detail

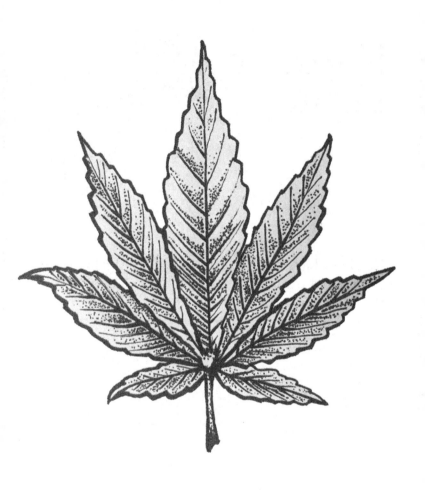

Indica
Relaxation, Body High
Couch Lock, Chilling, Stress Relief

Northern Lights

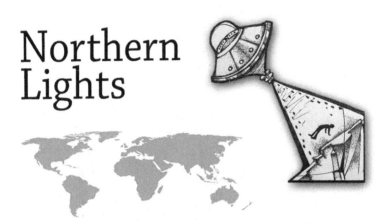

Northern Lights psychoactive effects settle in firmly throughout the body, relaxing muscles and soothing the mind in dreamy euphoria.

Cultivator... _____

Method... Flower O   Concentrate O

THC% _____   Edible O

CBD% _____

Top 3 Terpenes... _____
_____
_____

Notes: _____
_____
_____

Strain

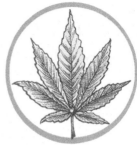

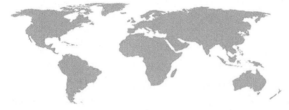

Cultivator... _____

Method... 🌼 Flower ⭕   💧 Concentrate ⭕

THC% ____   🧁 Edible ⭕

CBD% ____

Top 3 Terpenes... _____
_____
_____

Notes: _____
_____
_____

Mendo Breath

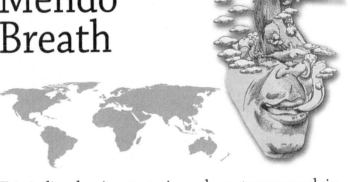

This indica dominant strain packs a strong punch in combating body pain and stress. The buds carry a sweet vanilla and caramel aroma. Recommended for late evening use.

Cultivator... _____

Method... Flower **O**   Concentrate **O**

THC% ____   Edible **O**

CBD% ____

Top 3 Terpenes... _____
_____
_____

Notes: _____
_____
_____

_____

Strain

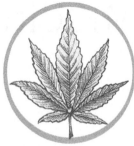

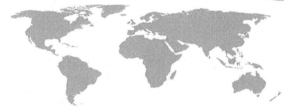

_____

Cultivator... _____

Method... Flower ◯   Concentrate ◯

THC% ____   Edible ◯

CBD% ____

Top 3 Terpenes... _____
                  _____
                  _____

Notes: _____
       _____
       _____

MK Ultra

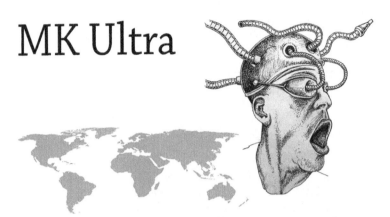

This is a very potent, indica dominant strain with heavy cerebral effects. It provides uplifting, euphoric effects in the beginning but leads to a state of full relaxation in the end.

Cultivator... _____

Method... 🌸 Flower O 💧 Concentrate O

THC% _____ 🧁 Edible O

CBD% _____

Top 3 Terpenes... _____

_____

_____

Notes: _____

_____

_____

_____

Strain

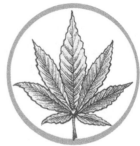

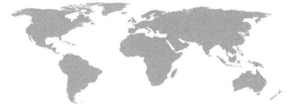

_____

Cultivator... _____

Method... 🌸 Flower ⭕   💧 Concentrate ⭕

THC% ____   🧁 Edible ⭕

CBD% ____

Top 3 Terpenes... _____
_____
_____

Notes: _____
_____
_____

_____

Strain

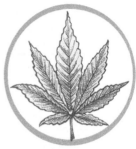

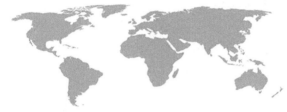

_____

Cultivator... _____

Method... Flower **O**   Concentrate **O**

THC% ____   Edible **O**

CBD% ____

Top 3 Terpenes... _____
_____
_____

Notes: _____
_____
_____

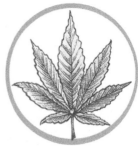

Strain

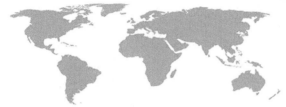

Cultivator... _____

Method... Flower ○   Concentrate ○

THC% ____   Edible ○

CBD% ____

Top 3 Terpenes... _____
_____
_____

Notes: _____
_____
_____

_____

Strain

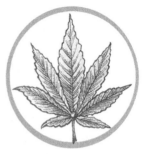

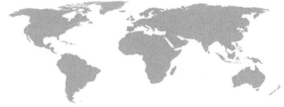

_____

Cultivator... _____

Method... Flower ⭕ Concentrate ⭕

THC% ____ Edible ⭕

CBD% ____

Top 3 Terpenes... _____
_____
_____

Notes: _____
_____
_____

_____

Strain

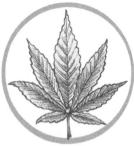

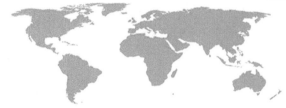

_____

Cultivator... _____

Method... Flower ⭕   Concentrate ⭕

THC% ____   Edible ⭕

CBD% ____

Top 3 Terpenes... _____
_____
_____

Notes: _____
_____
_____

_____

Strain

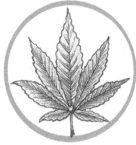

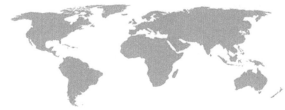

_____

Cultivator... _____

Method... 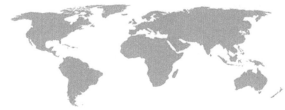 Flower ◯   Concentrate ◯

THC% ____   Edible ◯

CBD% ____

Top 3 Terpenes... _____
_____
_____

Notes: _____
_____
_____

Strain

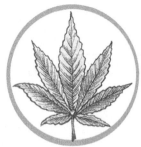

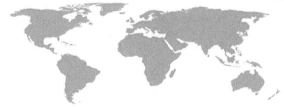

Cultivator...

Method... Flower ○ Concentrate ○

THC% ____ Edible ○

CBD% ____

Top 3 Terpenes...

Notes:

_____

Strain

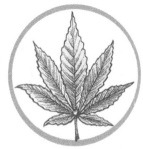

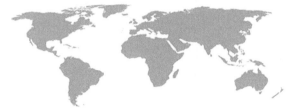

Cultivator... _____

Method... Flower ⭘   Concentrate ⭘

THC% _____   Edible ⭘

CBD% _____

Top 3 Terpenes... _____
_____
_____

Notes: _____
_____
_____

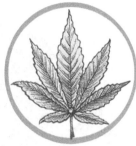

_____

Strain

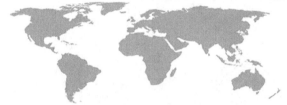

_____

Cultivator... _____

Method... 🌸 Flower ⭕   💧 Concentrate ⭕

THC% ____   🧁 Edible ⭕

CBD% ____

Top 3 Terpenes... _____
_____
_____

Notes: _____
_____
_____

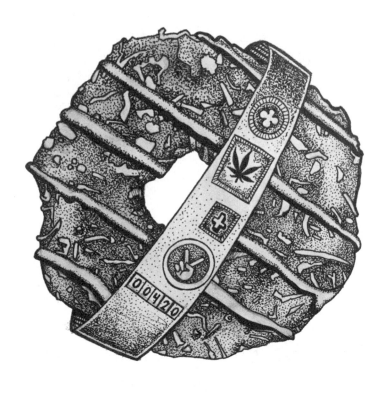

"GSC" Detail

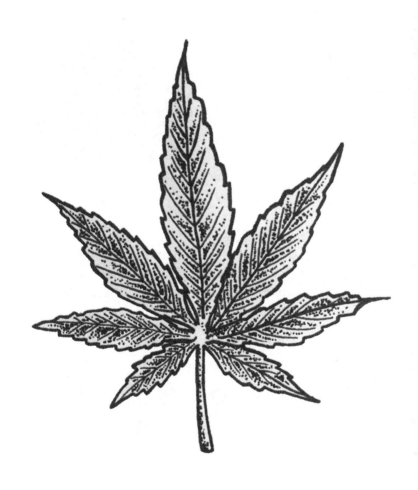

Hybrid

This strain contains the
best of both worlds. Sativa and Indica
Uplifting, Creativity, Relaxation, Stress Relief

GSC

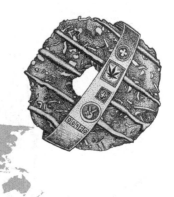

AKA: Girl Scout Cookies
This is a crossbreed of OG Kush and Durban Poison.
It provides a powerful, euphoric high with the
couch-lock body effects as well. Great for treating
anxiety, stress, and depression.

Cultivator... _____

Method...   Flower O   Concentrate O

THC% _____   Edible O

CBD% _____

Top 3 Terpenes... _____
_____
_____

Notes: _____
_____
_____

_____

Strain

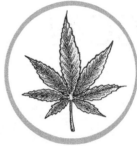

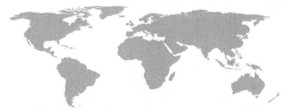

_____

Cultivator... _____

Method... 🌸 Flower ⭕   💧 Concentrate ⭕

THC% ____   🧁 Edible ⭕

CBD% ____

Top 3 Terpenes... _____
_____
_____

Notes: _____
_____
_____

GG#4

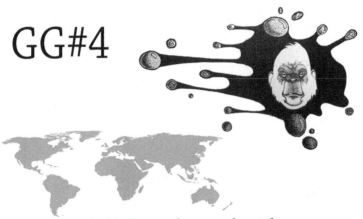

This potent hybrid provides just the right combination of euphoria and relaxation. Hence the name it will glue you to the couch. GG#4 carries a mix of pungent earth and sour aromas.

Cultivator... _____

Method... 🌸 Flower ⭕   💧 Concentrate ⭕

THC% _____   🧁 Edible ⭕

CBD% _____

Top 3 Terpenes... _____
_____
_____

Notes: _____
_____
_____

_____
Strain

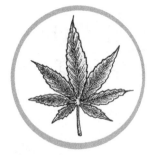

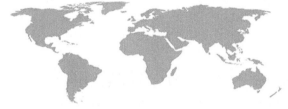

_____

Cultivator... _____

Method... Flower ⭘   Concentrate ⭘

THC% ____   Edible ⭘

CBD% ____

Top 3 Terpenes... _____
_____
_____

Notes: _____
_____
_____

Chem-Dawg

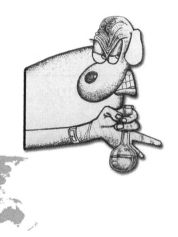

Chemdawg offers a very cerebral experience combined with strong-bodied effects. This strain is known for its distinct, diesel-like, chemical aroma.

Cultivator... _____

Method... Flower **O**   Concentrate **O**

THC% _____   Edible **O**

CBD% _____

Top 3 Terpenes... _____
_____
_____

Notes: _____
_____
_____

Strain

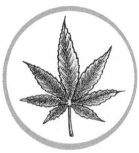

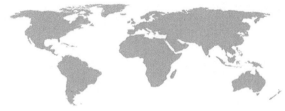

Cultivator...

Method... Flower ◯   Concentrate ◯

THC% ___   Edible ◯

CBD% ___

Top 3 Terpenes...

Notes:

_____

Strain

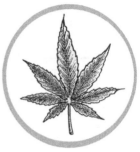

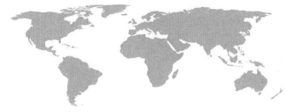

_____

Cultivator... _____

Method... Flower ◯   Concentrate ◯

THC% ____   Edible ◯

CBD% ____

Top 3 Terpenes... _____
_____
_____

Notes: _____
_____
_____

Strain

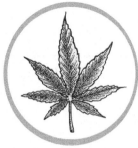

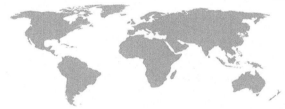

Cultivator..._____

Method... Flower **O**   Concentrate **O**

THC% ____   Edible **O**

CBD% ____

Top 3 Terpenes... _____
_____
_____

Notes: _____
_____
_____

_____

Strain

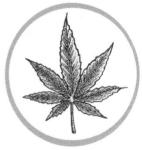

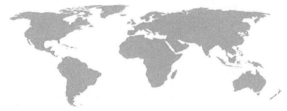

_____

Cultivator... _____

Method... 🌼 Flower **O**   💧 Concentrate **O**

THC% ____   🧁 Edible **O**

CBD% ____

Top 3 Terpenes... _____
_____
_____

Notes: _____
_____
_____

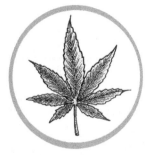

Strain

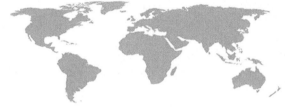

Cultivator... _____

Method... Flower ⭕   Concentrate ⭕

THC% ____   Edible ⭕

CBD% ____

Top 3 Terpenes... _____
_____
_____

Notes: _____
_____
_____

_____

Strain

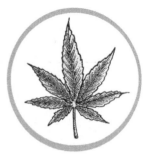

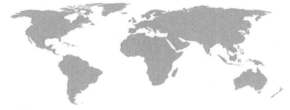

_____

Cultivator... _____

Method... Flower ⭘   Concentrate ⭘

THC% _____   Edible ⭘

CBD% _____

Top 3 Terpenes... _____
_____
_____

Notes: _____
_____
_____

_____

Strain

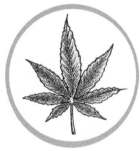

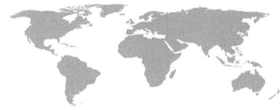

_____

Cultivator... _____

Method... Flower ⭕   💧 Concentrate ⭕

THC% ____   🧁 Edible ⭕

CBD% ____

Top 3 Terpenes... _____
_____
_____

Notes: _____
_____
_____

_____

Strain

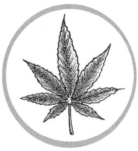

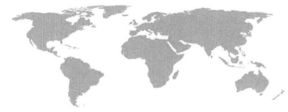

Cultivator... _____

Method... 🌼 Flower ⭘   💧 Concentrate ⭘

THC% ____   🧁 Edible ⭘

CBD% ____

Top 3 Terpenes... _____
_____
_____

Notes: _____
_____
_____

_____

Strain

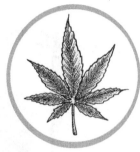

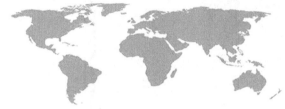

_____

Cultivator... _____

Method... Flower ⭕   Concentrate ⭕

THC% ____   Edible ⭕

CBD% ____

Top 3 Terpenes... _____
_____
_____

Notes: _____
_____
_____

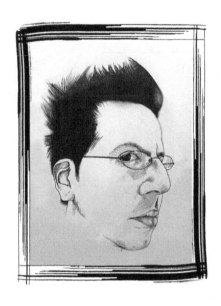

David is an author, artist, founder, and creator of Cochino, Inc. Born in Washington DC but raised in MD, he now resides in the Maryland countryside with his wife and two children. When he is not hard at work in the studio, you can find him providing his services to the Maryland medical cannabis industry. If you are interested in upcoming deals and future products, please give him a follow on
Instagram: *Cochinoinc* or
Facebook: *www.Facebook.com/CochinoInc/*

Made in the USA
Monee, IL
06 March 2020